Frequently Asked Questions

all about
antioxidants

RICHARD A. PASSWATER, PhD

AVERY PUBLISHING GROUP

Garden City Park • New York

The information contained in this book is based upon the research and personal and professional experiences of the author. They are not intended as a substitute for consulting with your physician or other health care provider. Any attempt to diagnose and treat an illness should be done under the direction of a health care professional.

The publisher does not advocate the use of any particular health care protocol, but believes the information in this book should be available to the public. The publisher and author are not responsible for any adverse effects or consequences resulting from the use of any of the suggestions, preparations, or procedures discussed in this book. Should the reader have any questions concerning the appropriateness of any procedure or preparation mentioned, the author and the publisher strongly suggest consulting a professional health care advisor.

Series Cover Designer: Eric Macaluso
Cover Image Courtesy of Barry Axelrod Studios, Inc.

ISBN: 0-89529-895-3

Contents

Introduction

As incredible as it might sound, it's true: Antioxidant nutrients can reduce your risk of developing more than eighty diseases, including heart disease, arthritis, and cancer; and can help slow the aging process.

Why are antioxidants so important? You probably know that people are more likely to develop degenerative diseases as they age. These diseases are caused by, or aggravated by, harmful chemical reactions that take place in the body. The process is inevitable—in fact, these same chemical reactions are what make us age. However, the good news is that these chemical reactions can be slowed, so these diseases are delayed for many, many years. For many people, the effects of these chemical reactions can even be reversed, enabling you to feel better and healthier than you have in years. The miracle workers in this process are called antioxidant nutrients, and *All About Antioxidants* explains how you can use antioxidant nutrients to feel healthier.

Antioxidants can reduce your likelihood of developing a multitude of deadly diseases, such as cancer, heart disease, and premature aging. Antioxidants work by destroying harmful chemicals in the body called "free radicals." These free radicals are the culprits in many diseases. Quite simply, antioxidants neutralize them. Knowing how to use specific antioxidants in the right combination can bolster your protection against free radicals.

Although antioxidant nutrients are in the news almost weekly now, I was the first scientist to describe them in consumer magazine articles about my research in 1971. I didn't invent or discover antioxidants, but I was the first scientist to demonstrate antioxidant synergism—that is, that antioxidants work together—and that a practical combination of antioxidant nutrients could extend the life spans of laboratory animals and prevent cancer. Today, we have numerous clinical studies that verify that this same protection applies to humans as well. The history of research on free radicals and antioxidants actually goes back to 1954 with Denham Harman, M.D., Ph.D. Now, more than forty years later, the evidence is unequivocal. The "take-home message" of this book is that you can immediately put these forty-plus years of research to your benefit now.

Do you need antioxidants? Among the diseases linked to excess free radicals are:

- Aging.
- Cancers.
- Coronary heart disease.
- Autoimmune diseases.
- Rheumatoid arthritis.
- Alzheimer's disease.
- Cataracts.
- Parkinson's disease.

If you are at risk for developing these diseases or have a family history of any one of them antioxidant supplementation can give you an edge and help prevent, reduce the severity of, or delay the appearance of these and many other diseases. In fact, one study found that the United States healthcare system could save $8.7 billion annually from reduced hospitalizations if Americans consumed optimal levels of antioxidant vitamins C and E, plus beta-carotene. The five-year savings would exceed $45 billion. At a time when the American healthcare system is nearly bankrupt, you would think that people would start paying attention.

As good as single antioxidants may be, one antioxidant alone cannot fully protect you against the many different types of free radicals. However,

a balanced team of antioxidant nutrients very effec-
tively helps protect against free-radical damage and
thus helps protect you from the different diseases
associated with free radicals. By the time you finish
reading this book, you'll have a good idea of which
antioxidants you should be taking.

1.

The Basics of Antioxidants

What exactly are antioxidants? What are free radicals? And how do they affect your health? In this chapter, I answer many of these basic questions. Generally speaking, antioxidants are good for your health, and free radicals are bad. Although antioxidants are abundant in fruits and vegetables, most people do not eat many of these foods and therefore lack sufficient antioxidants. As a consequence, supplementing with antioxidant capsules or tablets becomes very important.

Q. What is an antioxidant?

A. It might sound funny to hear that an "anti-something" is good for you. Quite simply, an antioxidant is a substance that protects your body and other objects from a process called *oxidation*. The best explanation is to think about why iron turns rusty or butter becomes rancid. Oxygen, which is essential for life, is a very volatile and reactive element. It reacts with iron to form rust, and it also reacts with the fats in butter to oxidize them and to make them rancid. A similar process occurs in your body. As you get older, more oxidation occurs—in a sense, it makes your body rusty. Anything that prevents or slows the oxidation process is called an antioxidant. Basically, an antioxidant protects other compounds against oxygen.

Your body produces some antioxidants (called endogenous antioxidants), but you must obtain others (exogenous antioxidants) from the diet. In fact, some antioxidants, such as vitamins E and C, are absolutely essential for life. The endogenous antioxidants are usually enzymes, coenzymes, and sulfur-containing compounds, such as glutathione. The exogenous, or dietary, antioxidants include vitamins such as vitamins C and E, bioflavonoids, carotenoids, and several sulfur-containing compounds.

Q. What is a free radical?

A. Free radicals can be bad for your health. Quite simply, free radicals are the bad guys that harm you, and antioxidants are the good guys that protect you.

Want a slightly more technical explanation? As you probably remember from your science classes, the basic or smallest building blocks of chemical elements are called atoms. An atom consists of a nucleus that contains subatomic particles, such as protons and neutrons. Normally, pairs of electrons orbit the nucleus, kind of like planets around the sun. Molecules consist of groups atoms held together by the actions of these pairs of electrons. Sometimes during chemical reactions, an electron will be pulled away from the rest of the molecule, creating a free radical. Essentially, a free radical is an unpaired electron. Free radicals are highly volatile and reactive, and they seek out another electron to make a new pair. Free radicals cause damage when they pull electrons from normal cells of the body.

Q. What qualifies a nutrient to be called an antioxidant?

A. To be considered an antioxidant, a substance must quench free radicals by donating electrons, and a little bit of the substance must go a long way. In other words, a few molecules of an antioxidant must protect many, many molecules.

Among the antioxidants our bodies make are the enzymes catalase, glutathione peroxidase, and superoxide dismutase (SOD). However, these are not sufficient, and we must obtain others from the diet. Some of the dietary antioxidants include vitamin A and especially the related carotenoid family of compounds, vitamin C, and vitamin E. Minerals are not by themselves antioxidants, but several minerals can become vital components of antioxidant enzymes made by the body. These minerals include selenium, which is needed to make the glutathione peroxidases; iron, which is needed for catalase; and manganese, copper, and zinc, which are needed for SOD. Sulfur compounds, such as the sulfur-containing amino acids cysteine and methionine, help the body produce the most ubiquitous antioxidant within cells, glutathione. Antioxidant coenzymes, such as NADH (nicotinamide adenine dinucleotide), coenzyme Q_{10}, and alpha-lipoic acid, are made by the body and obtained through the diet.

Q. What do the endogenous antioxidants do?

A. The antioxidants your body makes have very specific roles. Many of them are enzymes or coenzymes, which catalyze reactions in the body. The most called-upon endogenous antioxidant is glutathione, which is the primary antioxidant protector within your body's cells. Glutathione is a small sulfur-containing compound that teams up with selenium-containing enzymes called glutathione peroxidases. Other heavy-duty endogenous antioxidants are the superoxide dismutases. One type of SOD contains the minerals copper and zinc, while another type contains the mineral manganese. SODs specifically break up a harmful form of oxygen called superoxide into hydrogen peroxide. While hydrogen peroxide can damage cell components, it is not as destructive as superoxide. Another endogenous antioxidant called catalase contains the mineral iron. Catalase breaks down hydrogen peroxide into water. The selenium-containing glutathione peroxidases can also convert hydrogen peroxide into water.

Q. What do the exogenous, or dietary, antioxidants do?

A. The exogenous antioxidant nutrients are broader in their protective actions. For example, vitamin E resides in fat-containing body components, such as cell membranes and lipoproteins (such as cholesterol), and protects against many different types of oxidants. Vitamin C is the most important antioxidant in the bloodstream. Vitamin E is called a fat-soluble vitamin because it is compatible with fats, whereas vitamin C is called a water-soluble vitamin because it is compatible with water. Any of these individual antioxidants are beneficial to health. But they offer greater benefits when taken as a group. This is a key point I'll come back to over and over again in this book.

Q. How were the many health benefits of antioxidant nutrients discovered?

A. Vitamin E was once believed to be a vitamin without deficiency symptoms. It was known to be a powerful natural antioxidant, but no one could figure out how it worked in the body. It did not appear to be involved in enzymatic reactions or to be incorporated into structural components. This vitamin was a mystery that caused many nutritionists to be skeptical that it was indeed essential for humans. Little more was known about it, other than that it was required for the birth of animals. Without vitamin E, laboratory animals would resorb the fetuses before birth.

Thanks to the research on antioxidants and their effects on aging and cancer, scientists began looking at many of the nutrients anew in terms of their antioxidant activities. Studies of antioxidants' effects on the aging process led to the discovery that antioxidant nutrients offered protection against cancer. As an example, I presented my research on antioxidant synergism and life extension of laboratory animals at the annual meeting of the Gerontological Society in 1970. Some scientists felt that life expectancy was not directly extended, but that it was indirectly extended by preventing or delaying diseases, such as cancer. This was an interesting concept and my later studies established that this was indeed part of the explanation of the improved life spans.

Later, scientists began studying the incidence of various diseases among groups of people in relation to their intakes of dietary antioxidant nutrients. When I studied the incidence of heart disease in relation to intake of dietary vitamin E, I found that the more vitamin E consumed and the longer that those higher amounts were consumed, the more the incidence of heart disease decreased. Gladys Block, Ph.D., of the University of California conducted several studies in which she found that vitamin C and carotenoids were associated with reduced risk of several cancers. In 1993, Harvard researchers published studies showing that vitamin E supplements taken for more than two years were associated with reduced incidence of heart disease.

As people began taking more antioxidant supplements, they reported improvements in conditions ranging from menopause to arthritis. These reports, coupled with the development of plausible theoretical explanations, encouraged more scientists to investigate the possible relationships. Eventually, scientists felt sufficiently comfortable to study the relationship of antioxidants and the incidence of Alzheimer's disease, cataracts, and other disorders.

Q. What are some of the most common antioxidant nutrients?

A. The best known ones are probably vitamins C and E. Beta-carotene, lutein, and lycopene are part of the family of antioxidant carotenoids, found in fruits and vegetables. Flavonoids, another group of antioxidant nutrients, are also found in fruits and vegetables. Selenium, an essential mineral, is necessary for the body to produce glutathione peroxidase, another antioxidant. Some antioxidants, such as coenzyme Q_{10} and alpha-lipoic acid, are found in foods and also produced by the body.

Q. Which is the best antioxidant?

A. When people start debating which antioxidant is most important or powerful, they are missing the idea that antioxidants work together in concert. It is like arguing which link in a chain is most important. The chain is as strong as its weakest link. The same is true with antioxidants. There are reasons for this. Different antioxidants protect against different types of free radicals in different parts of cells and in different places in the body. In addition, antioxidants help each other like members of a sports team. This is what I mean by antioxidant synergism—the sum is greater than the parts.

Q. Would you explain more about antioxidant synergism?

A. I coined the term in the mid-1960s to explain what I was seeing in my laboratory experiments, and it later became the focus of my 1970 and 1972 patent applications. Essentially, antioxidant synergism is when the effects of combining antioxidants are greater than you would expect from adding up the effects of all the antioxidants individually.

This concept has become important in nutrition

to establish the teamwork effects of nutrients in general, but especially of antioxidants. Antioxidants should not be thought of as individual compounds. They should be thought of as complementary players on a team, or in the way that individual instruments form an orchestra. Doesn't a fifty-piece ensemble of various woodwinds, brass, and strings sound better than a fifty-piece ensemble of snare drums? Don't you think that a baseball team consisting of various infielders, outfielders, pitchers, and catchers would be more effective than another team of nine players, all of which are first-basemen standing around first base?

At first, I could not adequately explain the antioxidant synergism that I was observing, but some of the mechanisms were clarified with experiments. Now they all seem to be understood. Dr. Denham Harman of the University of Nebraska had experimented with single compounds to see if they had a protective effect. His first experiments were with sulfur compounds known to be protective against the effects of radiation on the body. In 1968, Dr. Harman demonstrated that a diet consisting of 0.5 percent of vitamin E increased the life spans of mice by about 5 percent. Soon after, I reported that synergistic combinations of antioxidant nutrients were more protective—with a 30-percent increase in average life span at lower and practical dietary levels. Al Tappel, Ph.D., of the University of California at Davis confirmed the biological synergism of the antioxidant nutrients used in my laboratory animal studies. The reason for the synergism is that some antioxidants are more effective against some free radicals, whereas other antioxidants are more effective against other free radicals. Synergism makes every link in the chain strong.

Q. Don't antioxidants also regenerate or recycle other antioxidants?

A. That's correct. Lester Packer, Ph.D., of the University of California, Berkeley, discovered that some antioxidants can regenerate other antioxidants, and this is another reason why they are synergistic. To explain a little more, after an antioxidant neutralizes a free radical, the antioxidant becomes a weak free radical. Another antioxidant can help regenerate this "used up" antioxidant. For example, both alpha-lipoic acid and Pycnogenol can regenerate used vitamin C, which in turn, can regenerate used vitamin E. This means that alpha-lipoic acid and Pycnogenol extend the usefulness of vitamins C and E.

Q. In what foods are antioxidant nutrients found?

A. A varied diet containing at least five generous servings daily of fruits and vegetables forms the foundation of an antioxidant-rich diet. There are thousands of antioxidant nutrients that occur in whole, unrefined foods that are not available in supplements. Unfortunately, many of the antioxidant nutrients are removed during food processing. Vitamin E is stripped from vegetable oils in the refining process and from whole grains during their refinement into white flour. Bioflavonoids taste bitter, so they are often removed from refined foods. While a diet rich in fruits and vegetables is the foundation, supplements are required to achieve the optimal levels of these antioxidant nutrients.

Carotenoids, another family of antioxidants, are found in the yellow, orange, and red fruits and vegetables, and in some greens. Bioflavonoids are found in most fruits, but particularly the blue and purple ones (such as grapes and blueberries). Vitamin C is found in citrus fruits, and bioflavonoids are found in the rinds (skins) of citrus. Vitamin E is found in whole grains, nuts, and vegetable oils. Selenium is found in whole grains, garlic, and Brazil nuts—if there is enough selenium in the soils in which they are grown. So, even eating a diet containing the correct foods doesn't guarantee that you will get optimal amounts of selenium.

Q. Who discovered that free radicals caused body damage?

A. In 1954, Dr. Denham Harman was the first scientist to theorize that the aging process was caused by free radicals. Until then, free radicals were thought to exist only outside the body. The only scientists that were familiar with free radicals were organic chemists who utilized the production of free radicals to help synthesize new compounds or make commercial processes for the production of complicated chemicals.

Harman was very familiar with both free radicals and the human body. He was a scientist experienced in radiation chemistry while at the Shell Development Company and a physician at the Donner Laboratory of Medical Physics on the Berkeley campus of the University of California. This unique combination gave him the background to have the brilliant insight that free radicals existed in the body and could cause damage.

The discovery of biological free radicals and the damage they cause in living systems is worthy of a

Nobel prize. This discovery has led to many advances in helping people live better longer. By applying the knowledge stemming from Harman's research, we have been able to delay many of the deleterious effects of aging, reduce cancer and heart disease incidence, and relieve much suffering. This fact is often overlooked as the tag given to Harman is "the father of the free-radical theory of aging." Unfortunately, the "aging" focus is too narrow and has obscured the broader implications of Harman's research.

In 1968, Dr. Harman demonstrated that a diet consisting of 0.5 percent of vitamin E increased the life spans of mice by about 5 percent. Soon after, I reported that synergistic combinations of antioxidant nutrients were more protective.

Q. How often do free radicals attack body components?

A. All the time! Bruce Ames, Ph.D., of the University of California at Berkeley estimates that every single one of your body's cells (and you have trillions of them) suffers about 10,000 free-radical "hits" per day. Much of this damage is done to your deoxyribonucleic acid (DNA), or genetic material. One of the consequences is that the mutation rate increases. Elderly persons have nine times the frequency of cell mutations as do infants. These mutations increase the risk of cancer. In addition, cell membranes, proteins, and fats are also being damaged by free radicals. Over a typical seventy-year life span, the body generates an estimated seventeen tons of free radicals. Your body needs to have its antioxidant defenses optimized at all times.

Q. What kinds of damage do free radicals cause?

A. Free radicals can damage all types of substances and tissues in the body. The easiest damage, and thus the most frequent, is to body fats. This is because fats are especially prone to oxidation. Scientists use the term "lipid peroxidation" to describe oxidized fats in the body. Lipid peroxidation sets off a chain reaction that will continue throughout the fatty material until stopped by an antioxidant.

Free radicals can damage the nucleic acid bases (adenine, thymine, guanine, and cytosine), which together form DNA. This damage prevents DNA from accurately replicating itself. Damaged, or mutated, DNA leads to the replication of incorrect biological information—such as cancer cells.

Free radicals can also damage proteins, meaning

that some body components may not function efficiently. For example, free radicals can damage the collagen proteins in skin, leading to tougher skin. Damaged enzymes (which are proteins) will not work as efficiently to drive biochemical reactions. Nor will the repaired enzymes be able to repair as much free-radical damage, and a downward spiral causes a snowballing effect leading to faster aging and possibly cancer.

Q. How can free radicals cause cancer?

A. There are several ways free radicals can cause cancer. I'll discuss them in more detail in Chapter 3, but here are some brief explanations.

- Free radicals can damage DNA, which causes mutations. Mutated cells can develop into cancer.

- Free radicals can activate so-called cancer genes, also known as oncogenes.

- Free radicals can suppress the immune system, inactivating the body's defense against cancer.

- Free radicals can activate carcinogens or "precarcinogens" to start the chemical reactions that lead to cancer.

- Free radicals can damage cell membranes and inactivate the sensory mechanisms that limit abnormal cell growth and reproduction.

By quenching free radicals, antioxidant nutrients protect against these undesirable activities.

Q. How do free radicals cause heart disease?

A. Free radicals damage the particles that carry cholesterol in the blood and, in a sense, turn "good" cholesterol "bad." This damage changes the cholesterol carrier in such a way that it enters into the wall of the arteries and starts the process that results in cholesterol deposits. Free radicals can also turn on blood platelet cells, which can form abnormal clots and set the stage for a heart attack. Free radicals can damage the lining of the arteries, which can lead to cholesterol deposits forming. The process is far more complicated than the old theories about eating too much cholesterol or fats. I'll discuss it more in the next chapter.

Q. Can free radicals cause arthritis?

A. They can certainly aggravate arthritic symptoms. Arthritis is characterized by inflammation. Inflammation usually involves "superoxide anion" free radical. Arthritis can be treated by reducing inflammation with antioxidants, including SOD. Several studies have shown that dietary antioxidants reduce the severity of existing arthritis. One of the promising antiinflammatory antioxidants is Pycnogenol, found in French Maritime pine bark.

Q. How do free radicals cause cataracts?

A. Cataracts are caused by free radicals reacting with the proteins in the eye lens. The eye lens is normally clear, so light can pass through it. Sunlight also includes ultraviolet rays, which generate free radicals when they react with proteins in the lens. These free radicals, if not quenched by antioxidants, damage the proteins in the eye. The damaged proteins are not clear, but cloudy, forming a cataract. Thus, cataracts can be caused by over-exposure to sunlight. High glucose (blood sugar) levels also generate free radicals and can damage the lens. Antioxidants prevent this damage by terminating free radicals. But because there are no blood vessels in the lens, the fluid around it has to contain sufficient antioxidants.

Q. Are any free-radical reactions good for us?

A. As strange as it might sound, we couldn't live without free radicals. The body uses free radicals to destroy germs. In addition, free radicals are needed for energy production. The problem is that most people are exposed to too many free radicals, a situation called *oxidative stress*, and this is not healthy. Antioxidant supplements help restore a balance.

Q. Can we control the production of free radicals in our bodies?

A. You can avoid things that either increase your exposure to free radicals or increase your body's production of free radicals. For example, tobacco smoke and smog increase free radicals in the body. Sunlight and x-rays also increase free-radical production. As the ozone layer in the atmosphere diminishes, we are exposed to more ultraviolet energy from the sun. Fats and sugars promote free radicals. Stress increases free-radical production. The increase in oxygen consumption required during heavy exercise increases free-radical formation. However, most of the body's free radicals are produced as side reactions during the normal utilization of oxygen to burn food to make energy. There are many things we can't control—you may not be able to move out of a polluted city, but you can compensate by increasing your intake of antioxidants.

Q. Why didn't we hear about the benefits of antioxidants until fairly recently?

A. Until about ten to fifteen years ago, there weren't too many scientists studying free radicals and antioxidants. When I began studying antioxidant nutrients in 1959, there were fewer than a dozen or so American scientists studying the role of antioxidant nutrients in aging, cancer, heart disease, and health in general. Today thousands of scientists are studying the benefits of antioxidant nutrients, and it's hard to go through a typical day without reading or hearing something about antioxidants.

This did not change overnight. It took the hard work of several scientists to inform the medical profession of the benefits of antioxidant nutrients. Also, until recently, nutrition wasn't taken seriously by the medical profession. Dietary supplements were frowned upon. Anything over the very low Recommended Daily Allowance was considered risky, and anyone educating the public about the exciting research proving the health benefits of supplements was called a "quack."

As more and more evidence was published, it began making the news. Doctors shifted their stance from "Don't take vitamin pills because they may harm you" to "Take them if you want, but they are a waste of money." Now, a high percentage of physicians take supplements and recommend them to their patients. At a 1995 meeting of cardiologists, about 90 percent admitted taking vitamin E supplements, though only about 75 percent prescribed them for their patients.

Q. Are there some general, simple recommendations for antioxidant supplements?

A. Jeffrey Blumberg, Ph.D., chief of the antioxidant research laboratory at Tufts University, helped found the Alliance for Aging Research to help disseminate exactly this type of information. At a press conference, this nonprofit research group noted that people could live longer and be healthier if they took daily supplements of vitamins C and E and carotenoids. They recommended that healthy people should take the following every day:

- 100–400 IU of vitamin E.
- 17,000–50,000 mg of carotenoids.
- 250–1,000 milligrams of vitamin C.

Dr. Blumberg reported that "We have the confidence that these things really do work." Later in this book, I'll provide more comprehensive recommendations for antioxidant supplementation.

2.

Antioxidants for a Healthy Heart

The common heart attack is due to coronary artery disease in which lesions (deposits of cholesterol and other materials) narrow the lumen (opening) of the arteries. The narrowing of arteries by deposits is called atherosclerosis, and when it affects arteries feeding the heart, it's called coronary heart disease. Since there's a lot of cholesterol in these deposits, many doctors assumed that cholesterol-rich foods would damage blood-vessel walls. But there's more to the process—levels of free radicals and antioxidants influence your risk of heart disease.

Q. What is a heart attack?

A. Having narrowed arteries (atherosclerosis), per se, does not cause the common heart attack. The narrowed arteries damage blood cells called platelets when the cells are forced to squeeze by. Platelets are the blood cells responsible for clotting, and squeezing and damaging them facilitates the formation of blood clots. The clots can lodge in the narrowed arteries, completely shutting off the flow of blood through that artery. This life-threatening condition is called a coronary thrombosis—a blood clot in a coronary artery.

When a blood clot shuts off the flow of blood in a coronary artery, the region of the heart fed by the artery is starved of oxygen and nutrients. The result is the death of these cells, which is called an infarct. This is the classic heart attack called an acute myocardial (heart) infarction.

Q. What are some other common heart diseases?

A. Another common form of heart disease is congestive heart failure, in which the heart is too weak to pump efficiently. Usually, the heart itself has enlarged as it has tried to compensate for the reduced output. Angina is the pain experienced in the heart when there is not enough blood reaching all parts of the heart during activity. Then there are disorders of the heartbeat rate regularity—too irregular (arrhythmia), too fast (tachycardia), or too slow (bradycardia) for an efficient pumping action. Spasms can clamp an artery shut and cause a heart attack even though there are no significant cholesterol deposits. High blood pressure (hypertension) affects arteries and is a risk factor in various forms of heart disease.

Q. How do cholesterol deposits form?

A. Cholesterol is a fat and not soluble in blood (which is watery), so it is carried in particles called lipoproteins. Two important lipoproteins are low-density lipoprotein (LDL) and high-density lipoprotein (HDL). The cholesterol carried by LDL is often called the "bad" cholesterol. LDL carries cholesterol to the cells. The cholesterol carried by HDL is often called the "good" cholesterol. HDL carries cholesterol away from cells. Cholesterol deposits seem to form only when LDL becomes damaged by oxidation. It's then called oxidized LDL. Oxidized LDL can infiltrate the artery lining and initiate a series of events that trap the cholesterol in the oxidized LDL, attract white blood cells, and form a deposit.

Q. How do antioxidant nutrients protect against cholesterol deposits?

A. LDL becomes oxidized only when the amount of antioxidants is insufficient to protect the LDL against oxidation. Oxidized LDL is a sign of very low antioxidant levels, because LDL is the medium that transports fat-soluble antioxidants through the body. The prime antioxidant that protects LDL is vitamin E, although other antioxidants help by recycling vitamin E. Other antioxidants can also destroy many of the free radicals before they reach LDL to cause damage. The tendency to form oxidized LDL, and hence cholesterol deposits, depends on two factors: the amount of LDL and the balance between antioxidants and free radicals. Both are important, but the antioxidant/free radical balance is the more important of the two.

Q. How do antioxidant nutrients protect against other causes of heart disease?

A. While a lot of attention has been focused on cholesterol through the years, the strongest dietary association with heart disease is a deficiency of vitamin E. Cholesterol deposits by themselves don't cause a heart attack. They are a major contributing factor to forming the blood clot (coronary thrombosis) that causes the heart attack (acute myocardial infarction). As long as the blood can squeeze by the narrowing caused by the cholesterol deposits in good volume, the heart will receive sufficient oxygen and nutrients to keep the heart tissue alive.

A critical factor then is to maintain the proper "slipperiness" of the blood cells and prevent a blood clot from forming in the coronary arteries. Vitamin E, and especially Pycnogenol, have a protective anti-aggregation effect on blood platelets, which are critical factors in the blood clotting process. They are particularly effective against the damage to platelets from stress and smoking.

In addition, the antioxidant nutrient Pycnogenol is a mild hypotensive (an agent that lowers blood pressure), which helps maintain a normal blood pressure. Pycnogenol also acts to maintain adequate nitric oxide levels so blood vessels can relax. Recent studies have also linked inflammation to heart disease. Antioxidant nutrients, especially Pycnogenol, reduce inflammation.

Vitamin E is important to the heart and arteries in more ways than protecting LDL from oxidation. As an example, vitamin E is vital to maintaining a healthy lining of the arteries. Tears in the lining of arteries are another way in which deposits can form.

Pycnogenol is a secondary factor in every way that vitamin E helps—this is because Pycnogenol regenerates vitamin C, which in turn, regenerates vitamin E. All of the antioxidants together form one terrific team to prevent heart disease.

Q. Can antioxidant vitamins prevent heart attacks?

A. Yes, they can—especially vitamin E. A study by cardiologists at Cambridge University found that daily supplements of 400 IU or 800 IU of natural vitamin E reduced heart attacks by 77 percent. This was a large scientific study involving 2,000 people over about five years. In many respects, this single study was the major turning point in making vitamin E acceptable to physicians.

Antioxidant nutrients slow or reverse heart disease. A mixture of the tocotrienol and tocopherol forms of vitamin E reversed the development of cholesterol deposits in people. In another study, researchers reported that vitamin E supplements, 100 IU or more daily, could slow the formation of cholesterol deposits.

Q. How do antioxidant nutrients protect us from stress?

A. When your body is under stress, your body increases production of the hormone adrenaline. Unfortunately, adrenaline activates the blood platelets so that they have a greater tendency to clump together and form a blood clot. While Pycnogenol can't make your causes of stress go away, it can help keep your blood "slippery" to reduce the chances of heart attacks and strokes.

Studies conducted in Germany by Peter Rohdewald, Ph.D., and confirmed by Dr. Ronald Watson of the University of Arizona, Tucson, found that Pycnogenol blocks the effect of adrenaline on blood platelets. Pycnogenol is particularly effective against increased platelet aggregation (stickiness and increased clotting tendency) caused by smoking.

Q. Does Pycnogenol work in the same way that aspirin works to prevent heart attacks?

A. Not exactly. Aspirin is widely prescribed by cardiologists to protect against heart attacks. The first studies showed that aspirin can reduce the incidence of a second heart attack in heart patients. Later studies showed that aspirin also reduces the risk of having a first heart attack. So far, this sounds good, but, unfortunately, many people develop serious problems with prolonged aspirin use. They can develop ulcerated linings of the gastrointestinal tract and an increased tendency to bleed. This can cause so much internal bleeding that it can cause death. Some people have been known to develop this condition suddenly and without warning. While aspirin therapy has benefit for many people, check with your doctor before taking aspirin on a long-term basis. In the Pycnogenol studies, the researchers found that 100 mg of Pycnogenol achieved the same desired effect on blood platelets in smokers as 500 mg of aspirin. Furthermore, due to Pycnogenol's effects on the enzyme 5-lipoxygenase, rather than on cyclooxygenase—the enzyme that aspirin inhibits—Pycnogenol did not increase bleeding tendency as does aspirin.

Q. How do antioxidant nutrients protect the linings of arteries?

A. One contributing factor in heart disease is damage to the lining (endothelium) of the heart and arteries. This damage can cause clots to form and allow cholesterol carriers to enter the artery walls. Researchers at Loma Linda University, California, studied the protective effect of Pycnogenol using endothelial artery cells. They found that Pycnogenol reduced the damage to the endothelium caused by free radicals. They also noted that Pycnogenol increased the levels of other antioxidants in the cells due to its sparing and regenerative effects. Other studies have shown that vitamins C and E also protect artery linings.

Q. How do antioxidant nutrients relax blood vessels to help prevent high blood pressure?

A. I'll give you a couple of examples. Pycnogenol has a mild hypotensive (blood pressure lowering) effect that helps prevent high blood pressure. There are two known reasons for this action. One mechanism involves the optimization of nitric oxide production in the blood vessels. Several researchers, including David Fitzpatrick, Ph.D., of the University of South Florida and Lester Packer, Ph.D., of the University of California, Berkeley, have studied this effect.

Nitric oxide has recently aroused much interest among scientists, after having been dismissed for decades as not being an important compound in the body—merely a waste product or inhaled air pollutant. Now, we understand that it has far-reaching effects throughout the body. Two enzyme systems control the production of nitric oxide. One enzyme system produces nitric oxide at a constant rate, while the other is activated by stress. Some nitric oxide is always needed, but too much can kill cells. Pycnogenol helps regulate nitric oxide in the body at optimal levels. It helps the body produce adequate levels of nitric oxide for necessary functions, while reducing the production of the enzyme that makes nitric oxide when too much nitric oxide is present. Dr. Fitzpatrick tested the effect of Pycnogenol on portions of the aorta and found that it improved the production of nitric oxide in the endothelium, which in turn had a relaxing effect on the aorta.

The other reason for Pycnogenol's hypotensive effect is its effect on dietary fat. In another study, researchers at the University of Maryland found that antioxidants can counteract the deleterious action of a high-fat meal on arteries. A high-fat meal prevents arteries from dilating normally. The ability to widen when needed is critical, especially in persons who have heart disease. In this study, healthy subjects ate a 900-calorie fast-food meal of egg, sausage, muffin, and hash browns. The meal contained 50-percent saturated fat. The researchers measured the dilation capacity of the brachial artery in one arm of each volunteer before the meal and again two and four hours after the meal. On the next day, the volunteers were given an identical meal, but in addition, they received 1,000 mg of vitamin C and 800 IU of vitamin E. This time, when the dilation capacities were measured, they were near normal, almost as if they had not eaten the high-fat meal.

While this vasorelaxation effect is important, Pycnogenol should not be considered a hypotensive drug.

3.

Antioxidants and Cancer Prevention

Cancer is not a single disease, but a group of many similar diseases. There are about 100 different types of cancer, and they all involve an abnormal behavior in some of the body's cells. Most cancers involve tumors. In this chapter, I'll explain what cancer is, how free radicals are involved in cancer, and how antioxidants protect against cancer.

Q. What exactly is cancer?

A. To understand the nature of cancer, it helps to first understand something about normal cell growth. Typically, the many cells of your body grow and divide in an orderly fashion. Normal cells also eventually die in a process called apoptosis, or cell suicide. When cells lose the ability to control their growth, they can divide quickly without any sense of order. This results in excess tissue, called a tumor.

There are two types of tumors, benign and malignant. Benign tumors are not cancerous and do not spread. Only rarely, such as with benign brain tumors, are they likely to kill a person. They can usually be removed through surgery, and they do not usually recur. In contrast, malignant tumors are cancerous—that is, they can infiltrate and destroy nearby tissues. Malignant cancer cells can also spread through the body and seed new tumors. Cancer cells seem to lose the ability to self-destruct—unless stopped, they just keep reproducing.

Free radicals are involved in cancers in a number of ways. They can mutate DNA, leading to the creation of abnormal cells. Recent research has found that cancerous tumors generate their own free radicals and promote still more mutations and abnormal cells. This is why some tumors always seem to be a step ahead of the treatment; they are changing rapidly.

Q. How does cancer happen?

A. Cancer is not the result of one single thing going wrong. A cancer forms through a series of steps. Simply having a mutated cell is not enough to create a cancer. The body has many safeguards to protect against aberrant cells. For example, the immune system can come into play and destroy mutated cells before they lead to cancer.

Free radicals seem to encourage the formation of cancers at many different stages. They can mutate, or permanently change, DNA so that it conveys the wrong instructions to cells—telling them to keep growing and not to stop. Normally, cells regulate their proliferation with their ability to sense the population of neighboring cells. Free radicals can damage cell membranes and inactivate the sensory mechanisms in the membranes that limit cell growth and reproduction. When cell sensors become damaged, cell proliferation and growth become uncontrolled. In addition, free radicals can suppress the immune system, inactivating the body's defense against cancer.

Based on research, antioxidants can stop or slow each of the steps in cancer development. Preliminary evidence suggests that antioxidants can also reduce the chances of metastasis and boost the immune system. Antioxidants may have a role in apoptosis, which helps eliminate mutated cells from the body. Although antioxidants seem to extend the life of normal cells, they appear to help cancerous cells commit suicide. These findings point to the fundamental regulatory roles of antioxidants.

Q. How do antioxidants protect against cancer?

A. Antioxidant nutrients protect against cancer in three ways: by destroying cancer-causing free radicals, by boosting your body's immune system so it can destroy mutated cells before they become cancers, and by reducing the tendency of cancer cells to adhere to other organs and glands. In addition, I believe that antioxidants inhibit several tumor promoters and the activation of some pre-carcinogens into "true" carcinogens. This effect has been demonstrated with antioxidants called bioflavonoids and explains part of their protective actions against cancers. Dr. David White of the University of Nottingham in England has reported that Pycnogenol inhibits an enzyme (monooxygenase) from converting the prime pre-carcinogen in smoke, benzo[a]pyrene, into its epoxide, which is a true carcinogen.

Don't sweat the details. Population studies have shown that diets rich in fruits and vegetables reduce the incidence of many cancers. Many scientists believe that the reason that fruits and vegetables are so protective is that they are rich in antioxidants, especially vitamin C and bioflavonoids.

Q. How do antioxidant nutrients boost immunity?

A. Several nutrients have been shown to boost immunity, thus protecting us from all diseases and increasing our body's ability to attack and kill cancer cells. Ranjit Chandra, M.D., Adrianne Bendich, Ph.D., and Simin Meydani, D.V.M., Ph.D., have been pioneers in showing that nutritional supplements stimulate the body's immune system.

Ronald Watson, Ph.D., of the University of Arizona, Tucson, specializes in studying the immune system and has conducted several studies with vitamin E and Pycnogenol and the immune system. In one study, Dr. Watson and his colleagues found that Pycnogenol boosted the levels of immune components called cytokines (formerly called interleukins), specifically the IL-6 and IL-10 secreted by T-helper 2 cells. These cytokines decrease during HIV infection and lead to progressive defects in T- and B-cell functions. It so happens that the same cytokines are also important in the body's resistance to cancer. Pycnogenol partially restored the decrease in IL-6 and IL-10 in laboratory animals that have a retrovirus very similar to HIV. In addition, Pycnogenol greatly increased the activity of a powerful type of immune cell called the natural killer cell.

David Hughes, Ph.D., and his colleagues at the Institute of Food Research in England have found that beta-carotene, found in carrots, increases the activity of white blood cells called monocytes. Beta-carotene does this by increasing the production of specific proteins on monocyte cell surfaces so that the monocytes can better recognize cancer cells. Beta-carotene also increases the production of tumor necrosis factor, which is a cancer cell killer.

Pycnogenol, vitamin C, and other antioxidants also protect immune cells from themselves. To explain, white blood cells release large numbers of free radicals when they are killing germs. Some of these free radicals kill off white blood cells. Antioxidants increase the killing power of white blood cells and, at the same time, protect them from excess free radicals.

Q. How do antioxidants reduce the spread of cancer?

A. Cancerous cells break off from tumors and travel through the body via the lymphatic system. They seed new tumors in a process called metastasis. Basically, the cancer cells stick to other tissues and form new tumors. This process requires molecules called cellular adhesion molecules, such as ICAM-1 and VCAM-1. Pycnogenol, quercetin, and other antioxidants reduce the activity of these adhesion molecules, preventing the attachment of cancer cells.

Adhesion molecules are also involved in inflammation, allergies, and atherosclerosis. By reducing their activity, antioxidants may protect against other diseases and disorders in yet another way. It certainly explains why antioxidants have been reported to ease allergic symptoms.

Q. Is there evidence that antioxidant nutrients actually reduce cancer incidence and death rate?

A. Yes, there is. Many epidemiological studies show diets rich in fruits and vegetables reduce the incidence of various cancers. Fruits and vegetables are rich in the antioxidant bioflavonoids, carotenoids, and vitamin C. In addition, there are hundreds of laboratory animal studies, including my own, showing that antioxidants reduce the incidence of various cancers. As far as human clinical studies go, there are a few. One joint United States/China study found that supplements of vitamin E, selenium, and beta-carotene reduced the risk of many cancers, including lung cancer and stomach cancer, as well as increased life spans. A well-controlled clinical study sponsored by the National Cancer Institute and led by Larry Clark, Ph.D., of the University of Arizona, Tucson, found that taking 200 mcg of selenium daily cut cancer incidence and cancer death rate in half, as well as increased life spans. A 1998 Finnish double-blind, placebo-controlled clinical study found that vitamin E supplements cut prostate cancer incidence by 32 percent. These are just a few of the many studies on the benefits of antioxidants.

4.

Staying Young With Antioxidants

Every living creature or plant grows old. As unpleasant as the thought may be, it's a fact of life. Yet some people age far more gracefully than others and look more youthful. This means that aging occurs at different rates, and research on antioxidants indicates that the rate of aging can be slowed. In this chapter, I explain how free radicals promote the aging process and how antioxidants can retard it.

Q. What happens to people as they age?

A. Aging is the process that reduces the number of healthy cells in the body. With fewer healthy cells, there is a higher percentage of unhealthy cells. Different organs seem to age at different rates in different people. When the percentage of unhealthy cells in a particular person grows beyond a certain point, the function of that organ is in jeopardy. In most people, the heart gives out first; in others, it's the immune system or brain.

The most striking factor in the aging process is the body's loss of youthful "reserve" because of the decreasing number of healthy cells in each organ. For example, fasting blood glucose (blood sugar) levels remain fairly constant throughout life, but the glucose tolerance measurement shows a less effective response with aging. Glucose tolerance tests measure the reserve capacity of the endocrine system to respond to the stress of an increased glucose load. This same diminishment holds true for the recovery mechanisms of other systems. Simply stated, the aging process is the body's loss of ability to respond to challenges or stresses. The mass of healthy active cells in each organ declines as a person ages, diminishing the organ's ability to function normally.

Q. What causes this loss of reserve?

A. By this point, you probably know the answer yourself: free radicals. The cumulative effect of trillions of free-radical reactions is the loss of cells. This damage occurs in a number of ways. For example, free-radical damage to the cell membranes can impair the cells' ability to transport nutrients into the cell and waste products out. As a result, the cell will die.

Free radicals also damage the cell's DNA, so that instead of replicating a healthy cell, it produces a mutant cell that does not function completely normally. Some of these cells may become cancerous, but most simply become less efficient with time. This cellular inefficiency is a hallmark of aging.

The result of these and many other types of free-radical reactions is that the number of healthy, active cells in the body decreases. This is analogous to the light bulbs in an old theater marquee that burn out one by one. For a while, the message can still be read, but as the number of burned-out bulbs increases, eventually the message is not discernible. In the body, the cells in each organ decline, but the organ still functions—up to a point.

Q. Can antioxidants help me live longer?

A. The answer is yes—but the real idea is to live better as well as longer. We should not want to just add years to our lives, but also to add life to our years.

In the laboratory animal experiments that I conducted, my antioxidant-supplemented animals lived longer—about 30-percent longer average life spans and 10-percent longer maximum life spans. Furthermore, they weren't just a bunch of old decrepit animals. They were healthier, looked younger, were more active, and had less disease. The question then became, "Will antioxidant nutrients do the same for humans?"

Unfortunately, we don't have double-blind, placebo-controlled clinical trials performed over the entire life span of thousands of humans to prove this—and we never will see such studies carried out. The expense would be astronomical. We do, however, have other evidence.

As the popularity of taking antioxidant supplements has increased, we have witnessed a decline in chronic disability, heart disease death rate, and, at long last, cancer. At the same time, the average life span has increased. Although this evidence is indirect, it does support the idea that there has been a positive effect on millions of people taking antioxidant supplements. Basically, if antioxidants reduce your risk of cancer and heart disease, they will inevitably extend your life expectancy.

There have been many other studies, in addition to those I described earlier. A number of years ago, I participated in a study with Linus Pauling, Ph.D., and Jim Enstrom, Ph.D., that examined mortality among health-conscious elderly Californians. This study found that the death rate was lower for supplement users. Male supplement users had a 22-percent lower risk of death and women had a 46-percent lower risk of death. Later, Enstrom and his colleagues reported that vitamin C supplements that provided over 250 mg per day reduced the mortality rate in men by 35 percent, which translated to a six-year increase in life expectancy.

One recent study, reported in the *Journal of the American Geriatrics Society*, found that centenarians—people aged 100 years or older—had substantially higher levels of antioxidants and lower levels of free radicals in their blood, compared with people between the ages of 70 and 99. They also ate relatively large quantities of antioxidant-rich fruits and vegetables.

Q. Can antioxidant nutrients help prevent cataracts?

A. Yes, they can. Cataracts, clouding of the lens of the eye, are associated with aging, with exposure to sunlight, and with diabetes. They are caused by free radicals oxidizing the protein that forms lenses. A number of studies have found correlations between high antioxidant intake and reduced risk of cataracts. One recent study reported that women who took vitamin C supplements—at least 400 IU daily for ten or more years—were less likely to develop cataracts.

Several antioxidants are of particular benefit to the eyes. Vitamin C, of course, and also vitamin E have been associated with a lower risk of cataracts. Lutein, related to beta-carotene, may also reduce the risk of cataracts. Lutein is the only carotenoid found near the lens. In addition, the lens is bathed in a fluid rich in glutathione. You can increase your body's production of glutathione by taking vitamin C, alpha-lipoic acid, and N-acetylcysteine—all very good and important antioxidants.

Q. Can antioxidants really create more youthful looking skin?

A. They can help preserve your skin, reduce the aging of skin, and maybe even reverse some damage. People with very weathered or wrinkled skin likely either smoked for much of their lives or spent a lot of time outdoors. Smoking is a major generator of free radicals throughout the body—that's why it has been linked to so many types of cancer. It's most visible effects, however, are probably on the skin. Similarly, exposure to sunlight's ultraviolet rays generates large numbers of free radicals in the skin.

To demonstrate the effect of free radicals, examine the skin on the back of your hand by pulling it away from the hand. Let it go and count the number of seconds it takes for the skin to spring back to place. Do the same test with people of different ages. In general, younger people will have more elastic skin that quickly rebounds compared with older people. Now, do the same test with skin from a part of your body that has not been as exposed to sunlight. See the difference? The skin is of the same age all over your body, but it has aged more where exposed more to sunlight.

To minimize free radical damage to the skin, minimize your exposure to the sun and don't smoke. To counter damage, take an antioxidant formula and consider applying an antioxidant cream or lotion to your skin. Antioxidants are absorbed and retained by the skin. Lester Packer, Ph.D., at the University of California, Berkeley, has conducted a number of experiments showing that skin antioxidants are quickly used up under oxidative stress. Vitamins E and C and beta-carotene reduce free-radical damage to the skin. Packer has also demonstrated that antioxidants in the skin work synergistically, which shouldn't be all that surprising because they work together every place else in the body.

Q. Can antioxidant nutrients help protect against sunburn?

A. To a certain extent they can. Sunburn is inflammation caused by free radicals, whose production was triggered by ultraviolet rays in sunlight. While antioxidants are not a sunscreen or sunblock, per se, they do increase the skin's resistance to free radicals and inflammation—and the skin's ability to repair damage. In a number of studies, European researchers found that supplementation with beta-carotene and the use of a topical sunscreen was far more effective in reducing sunburn than the use of a sunscreen alone. Other beneficial antioxidants include vitamins E and C and flavonoids, particularly Pycnogenol. Taking antioxidants internally, and applying them topically, can give you inside-out protection against sunburn.

It's not too late to take antioxidants—inside and outside—after a sunburn either. They will help restore normal levels of antioxidants in the skin, and they should reduce inflammation and speed healing. Remember that excessive exposure to sunlight increases the risk of skin cancer, particularly among fair-skinned people. It makes no sense to tempt fate.

Q. Can antioxidant nutrients improve fertility?

A. Yes, vitamin E, vitamin C, selenium, alpha-lipoic acid, and ferulic acid (an antioxidant found in Pycnogenol) have each been shown to improve fertility. Horse breeders swear by Pycnogenol and vitamin C. Antioxidants in general improve sperm motility—that is, their ability to swim. Many urologists recommend that their infertile male patients take antioxidants, as well as stop smoking. A number of studies in men have found that antioxidant supplementation normalizes the appearance of sperm and increases the likelihood of fertilizing their partner's eggs. In one study, 1,000 mg of vitamin C daily improved the sperm of men who smoked. Ami Amit, M.D., reported in the journal *Fertility and Sterility* that he gave 200 IU of vitamin E daily for three months to men with normal sperm counts but low fertilization rates. The men's fertilization rate improved by 30 percent.

Q. Can antioxidants improve arthritis?

A. Rheumatoid arthritis is an inflammatory disease. By now, you understand that free radicals promote inflammation. While antioxidants are not a cure for arthritis, they can reduce the inflammation, swelling, and pain associated with this condition. Vitamin E and selenium have individually and in combination reduced pain and swelling in arthritis patients. In Israel, a study found that 600 IU of vitamin E reduced the pain of arthritis in half of the patients, compared with only 4 percent of the patients receiving a placebo.

Arthritis may also be aggravated by low levels of vitamin C. When people do not obtain enough vitamin C, their blood vessels are more likely to leak. Some of these blood cells can leak into joints, where they stimulate an inflammatory reaction. Recently, French researchers described two patients with scurvy (a severe deficiency of vitamin C) whose symptoms included rheumatism. When they were given high doses of vitamin C, their symptoms went away.

Q. Can antioxidants protect against Alzheimer's disease?

A. Yes, they can. Free radicals are involved in Alzheimer's disease, and antioxidants have been shown to help. In a major study, published in the *New England Journal of Medicine*, researchers found that late-stage Alzheimer's disease patients who took 2,000 IU of vitamin E daily for just two years were able to delay for six to seven months key symptoms of the disease. It has not been proven, but I suspect that taking more modest doses of vitamin E (400 IU daily) much earlier in life will prevent or delay the onset of Alzheimer's disease. Ishwarlal Jialal, M.D., of the University of Texas Southwestern Medical Center said, "Anyone with a family history of Alzheimer's disease or heart disease would be foolish not to take daily vitamin E supplements.

One of the characteristics of Alzheimer's disease is the accumulation of beta-amyloid protein, which literally chokes brain cells to death. In laboratory experiments, researchers at the Salk Institute of Biological Sciences, San Diego, have found that Pycnogenol prevented beta-amyloid from accumulating in brain cells. I'm convinced that the best approach is taking a broad selection of antioxidants. I'll describe such a program in the next chapter.

5.

How to Use
Antioxidants

So far we have discussed antioxidant nutrients and what they do. We have put special emphasis on heart disease, cancer, and aging. This should be adequate to understand that antioxidants can indeed improve your health and help you live better longer. Now, let's put what we know to practical use.

Q. Why should I take vitamin E?

A. Vitamin E is the body's principal fat-soluble antioxidant. It's also an essential nutrient. No other antioxidant can really fit its shoes, so it is one of the most important antioxidants you can take. It's particularly important because of the huge amount of fats (particularly the polyunsaturated vegetable oils) people consume today in the form of fried foods. Such fats are very prone to oxidation, and they increase a person's requirements for vitamin E to prevent oxidation.

Of all the antioxidants, the evidence supporting the use of vitamin E is by far the most extensive. A recent study found that almost half of cardiologists were taking it. It comes close to being a "magic bullet"—a label given to it that was once criticized.

Q. Is natural vitamin E better than synthetic?

A. It certainly is. Vitamin E activity is shared by eight different compounds—four of which are members of the tocopherol family (alpha-, beta-, gamma-, and delta-tocopherol) and four of which are members of the tocotrienol family (alpha-, beta-, gamma-, and delta-tocotrienol). The most common form of vitamin E found in American foods is gamma-tocopherol, but this is because most of the oils Americans consume are highly refined. Biologically, the human body selects for the natural d-alpha tocopherol form of vitamin E over all others, though other natural forms do play important roles in health.

Synthetic vitamin E, which is identified by the term "dl-alpha" is not assimilated or retained as well as the natural form. For many years, natural vitamin E was rated about 36-percent more effective, on an equal-weight basis, than synthetic vitamin E. Two recent studies have found that it is actually twice as potent.

The manufacturers of vitamin E supplements prefer to use the esterified forms of alpha-tocopherol, which are much more stable than the unesterified form. The stable esterified forms are the alpha-tocopheryl acetate and alpha-tocopheryl succinate. Esterified forms can be found in both natural and synthetic vitamin E supplements.

Q. Can you explain a little more about tocotrienols?

A. Tocotrienols are a family of four compounds that have weak vitamin E activity. However, they may produce health benefits independent of their vitamin E activity. For example, preliminary studies suggest that tocotrienols can lower blood cholesterol and significantly reduce the size of existing cholesterol deposits.

Q. How much vitamin E do I need?

A. You certainly need more than the meager 8 IU or so found typically in daily American diets. The current RDA is 15 IU daily, and this is also far below the amount needed to reduce the risk of heart disease. The Harvard studies found that at least 200 IU daily for at least two years is needed to reduce the risk of heart disease. Based on various studies, the optimal amount seems to be 400 IU daily, though many people will benefit from still higher dosages.

Q. What are the benefits of taking vitamin C?

A. Vitamin C has many health benefits, but recent research has shown that large numbers of middle-class Americans do not obtain enough of it. The late Nobel laureate Linus Pauling, Ph.D., recommended vitamin C to reduce symptoms of the common cold. In analyzing almost two dozen studies on vitamin C and colds, Harri Hemila, Ph.D., of the University of Helsinki, Finland, found that 2 to 6 g daily reduced cold symptoms by about one-third.

Pauling also recommended that cancer patients take large amounts of vitamin C—10 g or more daily. Abram Hoffer, M.D., Ph.D., found that vitamin C decreased pain and increased life expectancy in cancer patients—but that a broader vitamin/mineral program worked even better.

In a study, Mark Levine, M.D., Ph.D., of the National Institutes of Health, found that the first symptoms of vitamin C deprivation were fatigue and irritability. In clinical practice, Hugh Riordan, M.D., of Wichita, Kansas, has consistently found that large amounts of vitamin C supplements relieve fatigue in patients.

Most animals produce their own vitamin C. Humans and a handful of other animals do not. But biochemically, they still seem to need large amounts of it. For example, gorillas in the wild eat foods containing about 4.5 g of vitamin C daily. Pauling thought that people need at least 1 gram (1,000 mg) of vitamin C daily—he took 18 g daily and lived to age 93. I think there are compelling reasons to take several grams of vitamin C daily.

Q. What are carotenoids, and are they good antioxidants?

A. Carotenoids are antioxidants that do double duty as plant pigments. For example, beta-carotene makes carrots orange, and lycopenes give tomatoes their red color. Their colors enable them to absorb specific frequencies of sunlight and prevent the formation of light-induced free radicals.

About forty to fifty carotenoids are found in the American diet, though only fourteen are absorbed into the bloodstream. There are actually two classes of carotenoids: the carotenes and the xanthophylls. Carotenes are hydrocarbons, meaning that they contain only atoms of carbon and hydrogen, while the xanthophylls also contain oxygen.

Beta-carotene has been the star of the carotenoid family. The body can split a molecule of beta-carotene in half to form two molecules of vitamin A. Since this is done only on an "as-needed" basis, beta-carotene is considered a safe source of vitamin A. Then it was discovered that beta-carotene was a very effective antioxidant, especially in protecting against the reactive oxygen species called "singlet oxygen." It also is vital to a healthy immune system.

In recent years, other carotenoids have gained scientific respectability. Among these are lutein and lycopene. If you eat a diet with varied fruits and vegetables, you probably get plenty of carotenoids. People at risk of certain conditions may benefit from extra amounts of some. I'll discuss this shortly.

Q. If I get a lot of carotenoids, do I need vitamin A too?

A. Many people have been taught that vegetables, such as carrots, are good sources of vitamin A. This is not completely true. There is no vitamin A in carrots or any other vegetable. Fruits and vegetables can contain lots of carotenoids, which our bodies can convert to vitamin A, but "preformed" vitamin A is found only in animals. Therefore, if you are a strict vegetarian, you may have trouble getting optimal amounts of vitamin A.

Many people will do better with preformed vitamin A in their diets. Vitamin A, of course, is an essential nutrient. Older persons and diabetics may have lower efficiencies in converting carotenoids into vitamin A. Therefore, it is a good practice to get some vitamin A in the diet, as well as ample carotenoids.

Q. What is lycopene?

A. Lycopene is one of the more important dietary carotenoids. The richest source of it is tomato sauces (more so than raw tomatoes); there is also some in watermelon and guava. One study found that men who ate ten or more lycopene-rich tomato meals weekly had a 45-percent reduced risk of developing prostate cancer. Diets rich in lycopene are also associated with a reduced risk of pancreatic and cervical cancers. Recently, a European-based study reported that diets high in lycopene have been associated with a 48-percent reduction in heart attacks compared with diets low in lycopene.

Q. What are lutein and zeaxanthin?

A. Like lycopene and beta-carotene, lutein is a very important carotenoid, and zeaxanthin, another carotenoid, is often associated with it. Lutein is found in many leafy green vegetables, alfalfa, marigold petals, and egg yolks. Zeaxanthin is found in corn. The body may be able to convert some lutein into zeaxanthin.

Lutein and zeaxanthin are essential for vision. They form the macula lutea, which, because of its yellow color, filters out harmful blue light. People with macular degeneration are often deficient in lutein and zeaxanthin and have only a thin, ineffective deposit of lutein and zeaxanthin in the eye. Because the macula is responsible for both "fine" and "central" vision, macular degeneration can lead to serious visual impairment and blindness.

Recent research indicates that lutein might also protect against heart disease and cancer. Because lutein is fat soluble, it is transported by the low-density lipoprotein (LDL) form of cholesterol. At least one study indicates that lutein protects vitamin E from oxidation in LDL. It may also contribute to the health of the immune system.

Q. What are bioflavonoids?

A. The term bioflavonoids, or flavonoids, covers thousands of nutritional substances that have a common basic structure. Nearly all are found in plants, which means they are also common in fruits and vegetables. The structure of flavonoid compounds makes them easy to donate electrons to other molecules, and thus they are usually excellent antioxidants. Although flavonoids have many similarities, they have differences, which lead to their varied biochemical activities.

Like carotenoids, flavonoids serve as plant pigments that filter out harmful wavelengths of light. Some common bioflavonoids include quercetin, rutin, hesperidin, genistein, diadzein, and those found in many herbs. Herbalists have been successfully using bioflavonoid-rich plant extracts for centuries to treat various illnesses. Flavonoids were discovered in 1936 by Nobel laureate Albert Szent-Györgyi, M.D., Ph.D. He found that flavonoids prevented capillary permeability, or fragility, which resulted in easy bruising and edema. Szent-Györgyi initially called flavonoids "vitamin P" (for the permeability factor). Later, most scientists dropped the vitamin P name, though flavonoids do have vitaminlike functions.

Q. What is Pycnogenol?

A. Pycnogenol is derived from the bark of French Maritime pine trees, and much of the product consists of a subgroup of antioxidant flavonoids called proanthocyanidins. Pycnogenol also consists of substances chemists call "organic acids," which are also powerful antioxidants. All together, Pycnogenol consists of about forty or so compounds. It is a good example of synergistic antioxidants. Lester Packer, Ph.D., has found that the key flavonoids in Pycnogenol are not as powerful individually as the total sum of antioxidants naturally found in Pycnogenol.

Q. What is coenzyme Q_{10}?

A. Coenzyme Q_{10}, or CoQ_{10}, is a vitaminlike substance made by the body and also found in foods, such as organ meats. Its primary function is in helping to convert food to energy. Secondary to this, it is a powerful antioxidant. These two functions do overlap. It is beneficial to people with various types of heart failure. CoQ_{10} increases the energy output of hearts, making them stronger. Unlike drugs, it does this naturally. Some cardiologists recommend as much as 300 to 400 mg of CoQ_{10} daily to treat heart failure, though most people do not need this much. Some recent research indicates that it may also help prevent the recurrence of breast cancer.

Q. You've mentioned alpha-lipoic acid—can you explain more about it?

A. Like CoQ_{10}, alpha-lipoic acid plays key roles in converting food to energy. German physicians have used it for years to treat diabetic polyneuropathy, a severe nerve disorder. It can also lower and stabilize blood sugar levels, making it important for diabetics and people prone to diabetes.

Alpha-lipoic acid is also a very powerful antioxidant. The body converts some alpha-lipoic acid into dihydrolipoic acid, an even more powerful antioxidant (which, unlike alpha-lipoic acid, is not sold as a supplement). In addition, alpha-lipoic acid can help regenerate numerous other antioxidants, including vitamin C, vitamin E, and glutathione.

High blood sugar levels generate large numbers of free radicals. These free radicals account, in part, for the complications of diabetes. Alpha-lipoic helps in two ways, by lowering blood sugar levels a little and by quenching free radicals.

Q. What is NADH?

A. NADH stands for nicotinamide adenine dinucleotide. This is a complex compound built around vitamin B_3 (niacinamide, nicotinamide). Like CoQ_{10} and alpha-lipoic acid, NADH plays a key role in converting food to energy. (These substances are not interchangeable—they function in different places during energy-producing chemical reactions.) Similar to CoQ_{10} and alpha-lipoic acid, NADH is also a powerful antioxidant.

Jorg Birkmayer, M.D., Ph.D., director of the Birkmayer Institute for Parkinson's Therapy, Vienna, has been a leader in the clinical use of NADH. He has found it helpful in many patients with Parkinson's disease, Alzheimer's disease, depression, and chronic fatigue. In one small study of Alzheimer's disease patients, Birkmayer found that 10 mg of NADH daily before breakfast for eight to twelve weeks resulted in striking improvements. The Alzheimer's disease patients' average scores on cognitive and function tests improved by 50 percent.

Joseph Bellanti, M.D., director of Georgetown University's International Immunology Center, Washington, D.C., recently reported that nineteen of twenty-six patients with chronic fatigue syndrome improved after taking NADH supplements. Eight of the patients benefited from significant relief of symptoms.

Q. What is glutathione?

A. Glutathione is the antioxidant workhorse within the body's cells. This powerful antioxidant is a sulfur-containing tripeptide formed in the body from three amino acids: cysteine (a sulfur-containing amino acid), glutamic acid, and glycine. Glutathione assists in keeping the immune system healthy, neutralizing intracellular free radicals, and detoxifying many harmful chemicals. Glutathione serves as a substrate, or chemical foundation, for many enzymes, such as the selenium-containing glutathione peroxidases that reduce free radical reactions.

Glutathione plays a key position in the antioxidant cycle, as it can regenerate most other antioxidants, but not NADH. Glutathione levels can be increased with several nutritional supplements, including selenium, N-acetyl cysteine, cysteine, and alpha-lipoic acid.

Q. What is NAC?

A. NAC, technically known as N-acetylcysteine, is another important antioxidant. It works chiefly by increasing the body's production of glutathione. A study by Italian researchers found that NAC supplements greatly reduced symptoms of the flu. Other researchers are investigating NAC as a cancer-preventing compound. It is similar to the sulfur-containing amino acid cysteine, but better absorbed and more efficient.

Q. What would be a basic antioxidant protection plan?

A. Fruits and vegetables are the richest sources of antioxidants. Therefore, the foundation of any antioxidant-boosting dietary plan would be to eat a variety of fruits and vegetables—a total of five to nine servings daily. Next, I would recommend a good multivitamin/multimineral support for basic nutrition. To this foundation, add the following:

- 200–400 IU of natural vitamin E.
- 250–1,000 mg of vitamin C.
- 50–100 mcg of selenium.

If your multivitamin/multimineral supplement contains these amounts, you're off to a great start.

Q. What is a more comprehensive antioxidant program?

A. Again, start with a diet containing five to nine servings of fruits and vegetables and a good multivitamin/multimineral supplement. To this, add the following antioxidants. You may be able to find most of these in a high-potency multivitamin or antioxidant formula. Strive for the dosages listed below, but a little less or a little more would be fine.

- 400–800 IU of vitamin E.
- 500–4,000 mg of vitamin C.
- 100–200 mcg of selenium.
- 15–25 mg of mixed carotenoids.
- 8,000–12,000 IU of vitamin A.
- 30–120 mg of CoQ_{10}.
- 25–100 mg of Pycnogenol.
- 25–100 mg of alpha-lipoic acid.

On top of that, if you're inclined and can afford it, consider the following optional antioxidants:

- 5–10 mg of NADH.
- 300–600 mg NAC.
- 5 mg of lycopene.
- 5 mg of lutein (along with some zeaxanthin).
- 50–100 mg of grape seed extract.

Q. Are all of these antioxidant nutrients safe?

A. Yes, they are. All of these substances are found in traditional diets, though many are removed, through food processing, from the modern Western diet.

Bear in mind that everything can be toxic at some level—including oxygen and water. The amounts discussed as being optimal are far below the levels that could cause adverse effects. However, it must be pointed out that selenium and vitamin A do have toxic limits that you should be aware of. Here are some upper limits.

- Selenium—Do not exceed 600 mcg daily.
- Vitamin A—Do not exceed 25,000 IU daily.
- Vitamin C—25 g and above may cause loose stools.

- Carotenoids—Take no more than 25 mg daily, if you are a heavy smoker or heavy drinker.

You may exceed these upper limits for short periods of time under the direction of your physician.

Q. What's the future of antioxidant research?

A. Thousands of articles on antioxidants now appear each year in scientific and medical journals. This is in stark contrast to twenty or thirty years ago, when very little research was being conducted on free radicals and antioxidants. Researchers are currently focusing on the most basic details of how they work—that is, molecular biology. This is about as "hard" as science gets. The evidence so far is that free radicals damage genes and activate "bad" genes, whereas antioxidants protect genes and activate "good" genes. Because genes contain the biological instructions for how our bodies work, this research demonstrates that free radicals and antioxidants function at the core of our existence. All trends point to future research being positive and confirming the many health benefits of antioxidants.

Conclusion

Free radicals and antioxidants are among the most important discoveries of the past 100 years. One can hurt you, and the other can protect you.

In the years since Dr. Denham Harman first proposed that free radicals fuel the aging process, researchers have documented their role in more than eighty diseases. All of the major diseases confronting people today—heart disease, cancer, Alzheimer's disease, and arthritis—are caused by or aggravated by free radicals.

The beauty of natural antioxidants is that they neutralize free radicals. In doing so, they can slow down and often reverse free radical damage—and reduce your risk of disease. And while many individual antioxidants, such as vitamins E and C, can have remarkable and rapid benefits, antioxidants generally work best as a group. This is because they are clearly synergistic.

As we move into the twenty-first century, antioxidant research is on the upswing. Thousands of studies on antioxidants are published in scientific and medical journals each year. Antioxidant supplements, which concentrate many of the antioxidants found in foods, are safe and relatively inexpensive, compared to the pain and cost of treating disease. It only makes sense to eat an antioxidant-rich diet and to fortify your diet with additional antioxidants.

The take-home message of this book is simple: Antioxidants can help you live better, longer—to add life to your years, as well as years to your life.

Glossary

Antioxidant. A nutrient that protects body components against undesirable chemical reactions.

Bioflavonoids. A class of antioxidant compounds produced by plants.

Carotenoids. A family of antioxidant nutrients produced by plants. Some carotenoids can be converted into vitamin A in the body.

Coenzyme. A cofactor that combines with an enzyme and helps the enzyme function.

Electron. A negatively charged elementary particle of atoms and molecules.

Enzyme. A biological catalyst that promotes a biochemical reaction.

Free radical. A molecule with an unpaired electron that can damage the body's cells. Free radicals promote aging and diseases.

In vitro. Referring to laboratory experiments performed in laboratory glassware.

Lipid. A chemical term referring to fats and oils.

Lipoprotein. A particle that is made of fats (lipids) and proteins. Lipoproteins carry cholesterol and fat-soluble vitamins throughout the bloodstream.

Nitric oxide. A simple molecule consisting of nitrogen and oxygen. Nitric oxide is a free radical.

Oxidation. The reaction of a compound with oxygen, or whenever a molecule loses an electron during a chemical reaction.

Oxidative stress. The situation when there is a serious imbalance in the ratio of free radicals to antioxidants. Too many free radicals and too few antioxidants lead to oxidative stress.

Platelets. Small blood cells involved in forming blood clots.

References

Clark LC, et al., "Effects of selenium supplementation for cancer prevention in patients with carcinoma of the skin: A randomized controlled trial," *JAMA* 276(24) (Dec 25, 1996): 1957–1963.

Enstrom JE, "Vitamin supplement use and mortality: Study that found no relationship is challenged," *Am. J. Publ. Health* 84(6) (June 1994): 1034–1038.

Enstrom JE, Kanim LE, and Klein MA, "Vitamin C intake and mortality among a sample of the United States population," *Epidemiology* 3(3) (May 1992): 194–202.

Enstrom JE and Pauling L, "Mortality among health-conscious elderly Californians," *Proc. Natl. Acad. Sci.* 79(19) (Oct 1982): 6023–6027.

Gey KF, "Inverse correlation between plasma vitamin E and mortality from ischemic heart disease in cross-cultural epidemiology," *Am. J. Clin. Nutr.* 53(S) (Jan 1991): 326S–334S.

Harman D, "Free radical theory of aging: effect of free radical reaction inhibitors on the mortality rate of male LAF mice," *J. Gerontology* 23(4) (Oct 1968): 476–482.

Packer L, "Interactions among antioxidants in health and disease: vitamin E and its rediox cycle," *Proc. Soc. Exp. Biol. Med.* 200(2) (June 1992): 271–276.

Passwater RA, "Slowing the Aging Process," *23rd Annual Mtg. Gerontol. Soc.*, Toronto (Oct 21–24, 1970). Also *Gerontology* 10(3) 28 (1970).

Passwater RA. *Supernutrition: Megavitamin Revolution.* New York: Dial Press, 1975.

Passwater RA. *Supernutrition for Healthy Hearts.* New York: Dial Press, 1977.

Passwater RA, "Vitamin E reduces heart disease incidence," *Prevention* 28(7) (1976): 66–72.

Rimm EB, et al., "Vitamin E consumption and the risk of coronary heart disease in men," *N. Engl. J. Med.* 328(20) (May 20, 1993): 1450–1456.

Stampfer MJ, et al., "Vitamin E consumption and the risk of coronary disease in women," *N. Engl. J. Med.* 328(20) (May 20, 1993): 1444–1449.

Tomeo AC, et al., "Antioxidant effects of toco-trienols in patients with hyperlipidemia and carotid stenosis," *Lipids* 30(12) (Dec 1995): 1179–1183.

Suggested Readings

Challem J. *All About Vitamins*. Garden City Park, NY: Avery Publishing Group, 1998.

Lieberman S. *The Real Vitamin and Mineral Book*. Garden City Park, NY: Avery Publishing Group, 1997.

Passwater RA. *Beta-Carotene and Other Carotenoids*. New Canaan, CT: Keats, 1996.

Passwater RA. *Lipoic Acid: The Metabolic Antioxidant*. New Canaan, CT: Keats, 1995.

Index